Atkins Diet Simplified

Definitive Guide to Concepts of
Atkins Diet How it Works

Esther J. Keller

Table of Contents

INTRODUCTION 4

WHY ATKINS...7

ARE THE BENEFITS OF THE ATKINS DIET SCIENTIFICALLY PROVEN?.8

ATKINS SCIENTIFIC RESEARCH EXAMPLES 8

CARBOHYDRATES AND THE ATKINS DIET 12

WHAT ARE CARBOHYDRATES? 12

ARE CARBOHYDRATES BAD? 13

DOES THE ATKINS DIET ALLOW CARBOHYDRATES?......................14

ALL ABOUT NET CARBS 16

WHAT ARE NET CARBS? 17

WHAT FOODS HAVE LOW NET CARB COUNTS?............................18

WHY YOU SHOULD REDUCE YOUR INTAKE OF CARBOHYDRATES IN THE ATKINS DIET.. 20

WHAT ARE THE BENEFITS OF LOW-CARB DIETS?............................21

EATING FEWER CARBOHYDRATES RESULTS IN MORE WEIGHT LOSS 22

WHAT IS INSULIN? 24

BLOOD SUGAR LEVELS AND THEIR EFFECT ON OUR BODIES................25

Insulin and the Atkins diet.. 25

Protein and the Atkins diet.. 28

What are proteins made of? 28

Proteins and glucagon 29

Fat and the Atkins diet.. 31

Saturated fats and unsaturated fats 32

How the Atkins diet works 34

Induction phase of the Atkins diet 35

Ongoing Weight loss Phase 35

Pre-maintenance phase 36

Life maintenance phase... 36

Why does the Atkins diet work?.. 37

Reduced calorie intake.. 37

Fat burning capabilities.. 38

Benefits of ketosis.. 38

Exercise and the Atkins diet 40

Benefits of exercising during the Atkins diet....................... 41

Follow the exercise plans recommended for the Atkins diet. 42

Metabolic resistance on the Atkins diet 44

How does the Atkins diet help deal with metabolic syndrome? 45

Introduction

If you're reading this book, it's obvious that you want to slim down and preferably stay that way forever. This is an admirable goal and the Atkins Diet will help you achieve it. The latest figures on obesity are very disturbing. According to a study conducted by the American Heart Association in February 2014, nearly 70% of American adults are either overweight or obese. This means they are at a higher risk for health problems like heart diseases, high blood pressure, stroke and diabetes mellitus. These figures have risen at an alarming rate over the past decade. According to the Centers for Disease Control and Prevention, after cigarette smoking, excess weight is the second biggest preventable threat to health.

The ideology behind the Atkins Diet is not primarily about losing weight. Rather, it is about maintaining a healthy weight. This is not just a diet; it is an approach to food that will help you to eat healthy for the rest of your life. Therefore, it is currently the most successful approach to weight loss provided the rules are followed closely. If you have the ability to do so, then you will definitely experience staggering success in losing weight. Losing weight is much easier than maintaining weight. Unfortunately, the vast majority of people perceive this as a short term effort. This is the reason weight loss is never permanent for those people who fail to make permanent changes to their diet.

This ebook has been written with the intention of briefing you in on what the Atkins Diet really is and how it works. It also includes a fourteen day menu plan to help jumpstart your weight loss. The Atkins Diet is spread over four phases.

Although, all the four phases will be discussed in detail, this ebook provides a diet plan only for Phase 1. This phase is supposed to last for a minimum of 2 weeks.

In a nutshell, the Atkins Diet is based on the concept that the body first burns carbohydrates and then burns fats for energy. Cutting back on carbohydrates such as pasta, bread, potatoes and sugar automatically activates the pathway that primarily burns fats. The result of this is weight loss.

You're in for many pleasant surprises as you read on. This is not your average diet of going after low fat foods and continuously counting calories, it is the one in a million diets which allows you to indulge in foods that not only tantalize your taste buds but also satisfy those hunger pangs – meanwhile improving your cholesterol levels, sugar levels, blood pressure and overall health. So, good luck and happy dieting!

Why Atkins

There are hundreds of diets available today which help in successfully losing weight. Then why go for the Atkins Diet? The simple reason is that the LCD 2.0 offers a big advantage: variety and taste. It doesn't require you to chew on carrots and cucumbers your whole life, all the while making mental calorie calculations; rather, it allows you to eat a variety of delicious foods in amounts that satiate both your stomach and appetite.

You may have heard many success stories of people who have lost weight the Atkins Diet way. You may also be completely convinced that Atkins Diet works. Still, a detailed account of the diet must be explained to you so that there are no grey areas regarding this approach to eating. In order for you to understand the mechanism of weight loss, we need you to understand a few basic concepts regarding nutrition.

Are The Benefits of The Atkins Diet Scientifically Proven?

True, the Atkins diet looks good on paper, and many people would like to believe it. However, many don't because it simply looks too good to be true. One reason for this is because many of the foods that are allowed on the Atkins diet are considered to be unhealthy and fattening. So, for an individual to recommend that you can eat all the bacon, fried cheese and meat that you want and you will lose weight instead of gaining weight - it's no wonder that many people are skeptical about this diet. To address such skepticism, scientific research is required.

Atkins Scientific research examples

There is plenty of research out there showing that consistently eating a diet low in carbohydrates causes the body's metabolism to shift from fat storage to fat burning. You will find research funded by prestigious health organizations such as the American Heart Association and the National Institutes of Health that show you can lose and maintain your weight loss by adopting and maintaining a low-carb diet such as the Atkins diet. This diet has even been credited with helping people deal with a number of ailments. Let's see a few examples of actual studies that have proven the benefits of adopting the Atkins diet.

- Research done by Temple University in conjunction with other scientific bodies

This is a study that was done on a small group of obese patients suffering from various ailments such as type 2 diabetes. When put on a low-carb diet for two weeks, these people experienced a spontaneous reduction in their calorie intake. This was followed by significant weight loss, balanced blood sugar levels and decreased cholesterol levels. This study was only done for two weeks and yet it indicated great results for the participants. Imagine adopting such a diet in your life for a long period of time. It's safe to say that it may help you deal with a number of chronic ailments you may be dealing with.

- Research done by the University of Kansas School and Duke University Medical Center
This research was conducted to see the benefit of low-carb diets on people suffering from Diabetes Mellitus. By changing their diet to a low-carb diet, researchers noticed that the subjects of the study experienced weight loss. They also noticed improvement in the glucose levels of the subjects, and in turn there was a decreased need for anti-diabetic therapeutic solutions.

These two research examples were based on feeding the subjects of the experiment with lots of animal proteins, low carbohydrates, vegetables, lots of healthy fluids and some daily multivitamins. They are just two examples of the many scientific studies out there that support the benefits of indulging in a low-carb diet such as Atkins.

The fact that you can solve health problems by partaking in this diet is a huge benefit. This means that this diet is not only for people dealing with weight problems, it is also for anyone looking to improve his/her health, as well as lift energy levels for improvement in the quality of his/her life

Carbohydrates and the Atkins Diet

The Atkins diet is probably the most famous low-carb diet out there. Most people think that to lose weight they need to reduce their fat intake. Fats have been blamed for a long time for weight problems when carbohydrates are the actual problem. This is why you will find many weight loss diets recommending the complete elimination or significant reduction of carbohydrates from one's diet.

What are carbohydrates?

Carbohydrates are foods that the body uses to make glucose, which is a source of fuel for the body. Carbohydrates are found in fruits, vegetables, bread, rice, potatoes, pasta, milk and milk products, as well as sugary foods such as cakes and candies. These foods are great sources of energy, but they also have a disruptive effect on our blood sugar level by causing it to spike. Your body needs balanced blood sugar levels to keep you getting a consistent supply of energy and also to maintain your well being.

Are carbohydrates bad?

There is a misconception that all carbohydrates are bad. This is untrue, because there are beneficial carbohydrates. The healthy or good carbohydrates are those that are high in dietary fibers and without added sugars. These are referred to as complex carbohydrates. In this category you have brown rice, fiber-rich vegetables, whole grains and non-starchy fruits.

These types of carbs are known as complex carbs because the body takes a long time to break them down into energy. This means that they give the body a consistent supply of energy, result in balanced blood sugar levels and help one stays fuller for longer. All these aspects are ideal for healthy weight loss and maintenance of an ideal weight. They also help to keep lifestyle diseases such as obesity and Type 2 diabetes at bay.

Does the Atkins diet allow carbohydrates?

The Atkins diet does allow the intake of certain carbohydrates, but in moderation. The carbohydrates allowed on the Atkins diet are the complex type. They are sourced from unprocessed foods rich in phytonutrients that are also known as natural antioxidants. These are mainly high fiber fruits and vegetables from which you will not only benefit from the fiber content, but will also get lots of minerals and vitamins as well.

The Atkins diet discourages intake of processed carbs. These are breads made from refined flour, pastries, cereals, pasta, white rice and white sugar among others. The amount of carbohydrates you consume is also predetermined. It is advised that the carbohydrates you consume make up at most 40 percent of your daily calorie intake; the rest must be proteins, healthy fats, vegetables and fruits.

By adopting a low-carb diet based on eating lots of proteins, you will find that weight loss is a natural consequence of your choices. It's hard for some people to limit themselves when it comes to eating carbohydrates. It is a delicate dance that at first may be taxing, but once you find the right level of carbs that you need, it's important to adopt the other requirements of the Atkins diet.

All About Net Carbs

When calculating the amount of carbohydrates you need on the Atkins diet, you need to figure out what Atkins referred to as the "critical carbohydrate level for losing" which is a figure of the most carbohydrates you can include in your diet while maintaining your weight loss during this diet.

Many people find that once they eat carbs, they can't stop. This is because carbohydrates, especially the ones that are discouraged, taste so good. To help people shift from a free carb diet to a low-carb diet a new category of carbohydrates known as "net carbs" has come up. Net carbs will help you figure out your critical carbohydrate level for losing weight when you are on the Atkins diet.

What are net carbs?

This is a recently developed category of carbohydrates whose aim is to help low-carb dieters get a chance to eat carbohydrates that they crave without having to suffer from the consequences of consuming too many carbs.

Net carbs are calculated by deducting the fiber content of food from its total carbohydrate content. What you get from this calculation is the amount of carbs in food that will affect your blood sugar levels, ergo your weight. The lower the net carb count of food, the better it is for you when you are on the Atkins diet.

An illustration of this is, for example, if you buy a packet of nuts, a typical label will have a calorie count like this:

- Total calories: 200 Cal
- Fat: 20 grams
- Cholesterol: 0 milligrams,
- Sodium: 20 milligrams
- Proteins: 10 grams
- Total carbs: 5 grams

You will find that the carbohydrates measurements are further broken down into grams and sugars.

For example, you may find the carbohydrates are made up of 3 grams of fiber and 1 gram of sugar. To get the net carbs of the nuts, you will have to subtract the dietary fiber measurement from the total carb measurement. In this case, it means subtracting five minus three. The result will show that your nutty snack has 2 net carbs. If it has sugar or alcohol content then, you will also be expected to deduct that, as well.

What foods have low net carb counts?

Foods that have a low net carb count are typically nutrient-dense and fiber-rich vegetables and fruits. These types of foods don't have a huge impact on the body's blood sugar levels. This means that your blood sugar will stay balanced, thereby helping you to avoid unnecessary weight gain. The balancing of blood sugar levels will also have a beneficial effect on your health, as fluctuating blood sugar levels trigger many health problems such as Diabetes.

Counting net carbs is easy, as you only have to look at the nutritional information of food. If you can't, the Atkins diet provides a carb counter that will help you to identify the nutritional information of any carbohydrate you want to consume. Adopting this measure will help you to identify the carbohydrates that work well for you in terms of keeping your weight in check and your blood sugar levels balanced, ultimately helping you benefit from the Atkins diet.

Why You Should Reduce Your Intake of Carbohydrates In The Atkins Diet

The calculation of things like net carbs seems intimidating. Many people don't do well with being limited, especially when it comes to foods. Many people also depend a lot on carbohydrates in their diet that it's hard for them to limit their carbohydrate intake. However, it has been proven that reducing your intake of carbohydrates can help you lose weight. So how do you do it? You focus on the benefits!

In low-carb diets, more emphasis is placed on consuming proteins and fats. While it may not be easy for many people to break away from carbohydrates, it has been proven that reducing the consumption of carbohydrates significantly helps in weight reduction. Focusing on such as benefits is one major motivation for you to cut down on carbs in your diet.

What are the benefits of low-carb diets?

You must also keep in mind that the weight loss from a low-carb diet is especially good because it gets rid of fats in problematic areas such as belly fat and butt fat. This is especially good because many people give up on weight loss when they find that fat in areas such as the belly does not budge easily.

You will also benefit from improved health when you reduce the consumption of carbohydrates in your diet. The stubborn fat that results from eating too many carbohydrates has been known to trigger dangerous ailments. It has been known to increase the risk of developing diseases such as Type 2 Diabetes, to triggering coronary ailments and even causing strokes. Research has shown that people on a restricted carb diet have less of these stubborn fat deposits to deal with. They are also able to significantly reduce the risk of developing such diseases in the future.

Low-carb diets have also been known to reduce the formation of visceral fat in the body. Visceral fat is the stubborn fat that leads to huge weight gain in people, as it is hard to budge. This type of fat can also cause inflammation in the body because it triggers the body to release hormones and proteins that cause inflammation. This kind of inflammation damages the body's vital organs interfering with the way that they work ultimately leading to chronic diseases such as arthritis.

Eating fewer carbohydrates results in more weight loss

All in all, what you need to understand is that reducing your carbohydrate intake will not only help you reduce your body fat, but it will also help improve your health. This is why low-carb diets are such good weight loss alternatives. These diets prompt the body to burn fat instead of storing it. When you don't give the body carbohydrates, which are its regular source of energy, it turns to the body's fat reserves for its energy source.

When reducing your carbohydrate intake, you need to focus on removing foods that have high-fructose sugars from your diet. Fructose is found in starch rich fruits, vegetables and refined foods. This is why you need to limit carbs, because even in healthy foods such as fruits you still find carbs that that can cause you to gain weight. A diet like Atkins will help you learn how to consume the right carbohydrates, in the right quantities so as to keep your insulin levels balance, your weight in check and your health at its best.

What Is Insulin?

Insulin and weight gain are two things that are almost always mentioned in one breath. Insulin is a hormone that comes from the pancreas. It is produced by something referred to as the islets of Langerhans. This part of the pancreas is responsible for regulating the amount of glucose or blood sugar that is present in one's blood stream at any one time.

Insulin ensures that your body determines how the body utilizes glucose from the food you eat. It can use it for energy or store it in the body in the form of fat for future use. In short, insulin balances your blood sugar levels. If your blood sugar levels are too high, you may suffer from a problem known as hyperglycemia. If your blood sugar levels are too low, you may suffer from what is referred to as hypoglycemia.

Blood sugar levels and their effect on our bodies

In the case of hyperglycemia where there is an excess amount of blood sugar levels, you will often find people suffering from Diabetes. This occurs when the body is not producing enough insulin to regulate the blood sugar so there is excess in the body. This situation also happens when the body produces adequate insulin but cannot utilize it as required due to one problem or the other.

In the case of hypoglycemia, the blood sugar levels are too low. Since glucose is the main source of energy in the body, when the blood sugar levels are low, you will find that energy levels are also low. In extreme cases, your body can even go into shock because it is simply not getting the fuel it needs.

Insulin and the Atkins diet

From these two examples, you can see that insulin is important in the body, not only for weight loss, but also for overall good health. The message that comes across is that you need to ensure that your blood sugar levels remain balanced to maintain good health and, of course, keep your weight in check.

The Atkins diet is great for keeping blood sugar levels balanced because it keeps you away from carbohydrates to a great extent. You are discouraged from eating refined carbohydrates such as white sugar, white flour, white rice, potatoes and other blood sugar spiking foods. Instead, any carbohydrates that you eat must be of a complex carbohydrate variety. When you use the net carbs calculations on these foods, you will also be able to reduce your carbohydrate intake more by shunning complex foods that have a high, net carb count.

To understand the correlation between carbohydrate intake and insulin, you have to realize that when you eat more carbs than you need, the excess will be stored in the form of fat or glycogen. If your insulin levels rise, it will prevent the carbohydrates from being turned into fuel efficiently, and will instead encourage their storage as fat in the body.

By limiting your carbohydrate intake as the Atkins diet requires, you will stimulate increased fat burning in the body. It will help you get rid of unwanted fat stores. It will also improve your metabolism. All these benefits will only be beneficial towards maintaining your ideal weight and keeping chronic illnesses at bay.

Protein and the Atkins Diet

Proteins are the building blocks of the body. Every cell in our bodies contains some protein. The body needs proteins to maintain itself by repairing any broken down cells, and also in the creation of new ones. Therefore, this food group is important for growth and development of the body as well as maintenance, which is very important since the body goes through a lot of wear and tear in the course of our daily lives.

What are proteins made of?

Proteins are made up of amino acids. Amino acids are found in food sources such as eggs, meat and fish. They are also found in plant sources such as nuts, soy, legumes and even beans. You will also find them in grains such as quinoa. This means that even if you are a vegetarian, you can get adequate amounts of protein from your diet. The amino acids found in proteins are found in three classes. There are essential, non-essential and conditional amino acids.

Essential amino acids as the name suggests are very important to the body. However, they cannot be made by the body, and are sourced from protein-rich foods. Non-essential amino acids can be made from essential amino acids or be accessed from other protein foods. Conditional amino acids are only needed in times when the body is not doing well, such as during an illness. Whatever the case, adequate amounts of protein amino acids are required for good health in the body.

Proteins and glucagon

Glucagon is essential in controlling the release of fat in the body and, therefore, can help increase one's metabolic rate significantly. An increased metabolic rate means a higher rate of fat burning in the body. Proteins are, therefore, very important in the maintenance of healthy insulin levels in the body and most especially in weight management. Studies have shown that diets based on high protein intake lead to more fat loss and health benefits than what is experienced in high-carb diets. Eating a protein-rich diet increases your metabolism, reduces your fat intake and increases your energy levels.

Although health experts recommend that one consume half a gram of protein for every pound of weight they have, this is not accurate in many cases. You should tailor your protein intake to the type of activity you engage in, and based on the kind of weight you are experiencing. For example if you are a weight lifter you need more protein than most average people. Your age will also determine the amount of protein you take as older people need more protein than younger people. Whatever your protein intake, you will realize that protein-rich diets such as the Atkins diet are very beneficial.

Fat and the Atkins Diet

Fats are despised by many people; some don't even eat anything with fat. So if you describe fat to some people as a nutrient, they will be skeptical. The truth is that fat is a nutrient that is very important for normal body functions to occur in the body. Fat is a great source of energy and it also enables other nutrients from food such as vitamins and minerals to be utilized properly in the body.

Fats are made up of a number of compounds that are soluble in organic solvents, but insoluble in water. At room temperature, some fats remain solid, while others turn into liquid form. The change in room temperature is determined by the composition of the fat.

One thing you have to understand is that you cannot live without fat in your diet. Fat is essential for supporting a number of your body functions. The composition of fats is what characterizes them as healthy or unhealthy or good and bad fats as they are commonly referred to. You also have to keep in mind that fat has a high caloric content. If you eat more of it than you need to, then it will definitely be stored in the body and lead to unwanted weight gain.

Saturated fats and unsaturated fats

Saturated and unsaturated fats are the names used to refer to the bad and good fats in food respectively. Saturated fats are mainly derived from animal sources such as poultry, dairy products, and red meat among other sources. This form of fat, when taken in excess, can raise the level of low-density lipoproteins in the body. This type of cholesterol can increase the risk of developing cardiovascular ailments and Type 2 diabetes.

Unsaturated fats are healthy fats when taken in low quantities. These types of fat can balance sugar levels, help in weight reduction and prevent heart ailments from developing. The Atkins diet allows people to eat a lot of fats when they allow people to eat animal proteins such as pork. Therefore many people are skeptical about the effectiveness of this diet.

This is where the secret lies. If you reduce your carbohydrate intake, then consuming saturated fats such as the ones allowed in the Atkins diet will not affect your health in a negative way. If you take saturated fats in combination with lots of carbohydrates, the carbs prevent the body from burning fat as it should. Hence, the fat deposits will keep piling up in the body. With a low carb diet you will find that most of the fats you take in are burned by the body to create energy for the body instead thereby replacing carbohydrates as your body's source of energy.

This means that you will burn the fats you consume when on the Atkins diet if you follow the instructions. Not only will you burn the fat you eat, but you also burn stubborn fat storages in the body. Your body basically turns into an efficient fat burning machine, helping you to realize significant weight loss in a short time, even when you are not working out frantically. This is how fats work into the Atkins diet.

How the Atkins Diet Works

We have seen how different food groups work in the body when it comes to weight loss and health issues. The cornerstone of the Atkins diet's success is based on its low-carb approach.

Dr. Atkins was fond of saying that carbohydrates are the cause of many of our health problems and lifestyle issues. This is true. It doesn't help that carbs are the cornerstone of many people's meals. They are loved, they taste great and they are hard to quit. The bottom line is that they are not good for our bodies. If you make the choice to cut down on your carbohydrate intake as recommended in the Atkins diet, you will surely benefit from it in spades.

In order for the Atkins diet to work, you need to follow all the stages required. It starts with the first point known as the induction phase. This is followed by the ongoing weight loss stage. The third stage is the pre-maintenance phase. The last phase is the lifetime maintenance phase.

Induction phase of the Atkins diet

This is normally set as the first 14 days of the diet. The focus during this period is to shift the body from metabolizing carbohydrates to metabolizing fats. You will also be working at balancing your blood sugar levels and dealing with food cravings. The other thing you will work at is to condition your body to burn fat without having to count your calories or work out excessively. Lastly, you will be expected to get your body into a "state of ketosis," at which the body has an extremely high fat-burning rate. All of these stages in the first phase of the diet will force your body to burn fat stores and also withdraw from your dependence on carbohydrates as you adopt this low-carb diet.

Ongoing Weight loss Phase

The second phase follows the first fourteen days of the diet when your body has learnt to live relatively well without the amount of carbs you were used to consuming before the diet. At this stage, you will be allowed to reintroduce carbohydrates back into your diet. You will have to eat wholesome carbs in moderate amounts. It is during this phase that you will discover the amount of carbohydrates you can consume without gaining weight known as the critical carbohydrate level for losing weight. At this stage, you will have attained your ideal weight and this will take you to the third phase.

Pre-maintenance phase

In the third phase of the Atkins diet, you are expected to adopt habits that will help you to maintain your weight loss in the long run. This will help you to cement the healthy eating habits that have helped you lose weight along the way.

Life maintenance phase

The last phase is the lifetime maintenance where you make the Atkins diet your way of life. Many people that have adopted the Atkins diet permanently are in this phase. By the time you get here, you will have completely adopted a low-carb diet approach.

Why Does the Atkins Diet Work?

There is no doubt that the Atkins diet works with good results, even if many people are skeptical about it. The question is why? How can a diet that allows people to eat as many proteins and fat foods as they want, especially animal fats, lead to weight reduction? Most importantly, how do people on this diet maintain their weight loss over the long term?

Reduced calorie intake

The success of the Atkins diet lies first within the low-calorie intake. Research has shown that people on the Atkins diet eat fewer calories than people on a low-fat diet, even if they can eat as much fat as they desire. This is because proteins and fats have the ability to act as appetite suppressants.

All the meat, eggs, and fish that people on this diet consume help them to keep hunger pangs at bay. Carbohydrates influence blood sugar levels, and thereby can cause hunger pangs. On the contrary, proteins have the ability to make the body feel like it is full even when small quantities of proteins have been consumed. You will see that people on this diet are not always eating

Fat burning capabilities

Regardless of the amount of protein and fat eaten on this diet, you can still burn more calories than you eat. This is because the body burns more calories when it is being fueled by fats and proteins as compared to when it is being fueled by carbohydrates. It takes more calories to burn fats and proteins than it does to burn carbohydrates; the result is that there is less fat storage with such a diet. This is why you see fats stored in stubborn areas such as the abdomen that seem to melt away when on this diet, whereas normally they are the hardest parts to slim down.

Benefits of ketosis

The other reason this diet works is the ketosis process. To understand what this process is, you must understand what ketones are. Ketones are substances that are realized when fats are burnt in the body. When the levels of ketones in the body are elevated, the body is said to be in a state of ketosis. When ketone levels are elevated, an individual feels less hungry. This symbolizes the body's switch from being a carbohydrate-burning organism to a fat burning organism, which is characterized by significant weight loss.

When your body is in a state of ketosis, fat become the body's main source of energy. This refers to the body's fat stores as well as the fats that you consume. When these fats are burned, the body loses unwanted weight. Although high level of ketones in the body can cause illness, in the Atkins diet any unused ketones are expelled through sweating and urination. In the Atkins diet, this is one way that your body gets rid of unused calories from fats and proteins.

In general, with the Atkins diet, you will lose weight and even eat less without much effort on your part -- as long as you stick to the diet plan.

Exercise and the Atkins Diet

The truth is that the Atkins diet is one of the diets that will require you to do very little exercise, as most of the weight is lost due to your diet plan.

However, exercise is not prohibited. In fact, you will find that the food plan you are given encourages exercise, and even schedules in foods you can eat to help you increase your physical activity. Although most people associate exercise with weight loss or healthy weight maintenance, it does more for your health and emotional well-being than anything else. For this reason, you are encouraged to include exercise in your day to day activities when you are on the Atkins diet, as it will enhance the benefits of the diet.

Benefits of exercising during the Atkins diet

There are four benefits gained by exercising along side the Atkins diet. By exercising throughout the Atkins diet, you will increase the fat burning capabilities of your body. Secondly, you will boost your metabolism. Thirdly, you will increase the circulation in your body and eliminate toxins in through your lymph systems and sweat glands. Lastly, it will have a good effect on your blood sugar levels.

Where do blood sugar levels and exercise factor in? Your body has to process carbohydrates properly to keep your blood sugar levels stable. If you lead a sedentary life, even with the changes in your diet, it will mean that any little carbohydrates you consume can send your blood sugar levels through the roof. The result will be insufficient weight loss, even as you are working hard to maintain the rules of the Atkins diet. By exercising, the body will use the carbohydrates you eat efficiently, and your blood sugar levels will remain stable.

Follow the exercise plans recommended for the Atkins diet.

The best thing about exercising on the Atkins diet is that it will help you to get better body definition and increase your strength. You will also strengthen your bones. Just losing weight and yet not strengthening your body is a waste of time. You need to lose weight, tone your body and strengthen it as well.

It is important to realize that since the Atkins diet limits the amount of carbs you can eat and this is the main energy source from food, you have to learn to schedule your meals in a way that will help you to have enough energy to workout.

You will find that the Atkins diet has exercise plans for each age group. These exercise plans are made for the young, middle-aged and elderly. You will see that the plans emphasize on increasing the percentage of fat you consume, so as to have more endurance when exercising. This is supposed to stand in for carbohydrates, which help you to endure a workout in normal circumstances.

You will also be expected to eat frequently so that you maintain a fast metabolism as well as your muscle strength. This, combined with a minimum of 30 minutes of exercise a day, will ensure that you burn a good amount of calories that will cement the benefits of the diet for you. Make sure you start small and increase the time as you go along as your body gets used to exercising when on the Atkins diet.

Metabolic Resistance on the Atkins Diet

This is also referred to as metabolic syndrome or insulin resistance syndrome. It is a problem that encompasses a lot of health problems that occur in the body, stemming from a problem with unwanted weight. People suffering from metabolic resistance have a higher chance of experiencing heart problems, strokes and diabetes.

Although the cause of metabolic syndrome is not known, many subscribe it to genetics. It is also thought that being overweight and physically inactive can put you at risk of suffering from this problem. People suffering from insulin resistance syndrome have excess fat around the abdomen, suffer from hypertension and have low levels of good cholesterol. They may also suffer from unhealthy blood glucose levels. If you have three or more of these issues, you might suffer from metabolic syndrome.

How does the Atkins diet help deal with metabolic syndrome?

The question is, how do people suffering from metabolic syndrome deal with this problem while on the Atkins diet? You also have to ask – can the Atkins diet be used to deal with metabolic syndrome so as to help regain optimum health and attain ideal weight loss. The answer is yes. First, the Atkins diet has been known to attack the stubborn fat along the abdomen and other areas of the body, which is one of the telltale signs of metabolic syndrome.

People suffering from metabolic syndrome have dealt with it using the Atkins diet because it helps to improve cholesterol levels. This diet also helps to lower inflammation and improve insulin levels in the body. Statistics also back up the efficacy of this diet when combatting metabolic syndrome. This is based on its ability to help the body lose calories, especially in stubborn areas such as the tummy.

The fact that this diet limits carbohydrate intake is great. Carbohydrates are seen as the biggest cause of obesity, blood sugar problems and cardiovascular problems. Even for people that are not suffering from metabolic syndrome, this diet also improves health significantly. The Atkins diet encourages people to eat foods that are filling, thereby reducing the calories that one consumes will definitely help deal with obesity..

This diet also helps one deal with maintaining stable blood sugar levels. The foods accepted on this diet promote a feeling of fullness and are also known for releasing energy consistently, which is something that ensures that the blood sugar levels in the body remain stable. With your diet in check, you will not have to deal with Diabetes, which is another trigger sign of this syndrome.

Many people think that since abdominal fat is one among the causes of this syndrome, eating a diet with lots of fats such as the Atkins diet may increase the risk of getting this syndrome instead of helping deal with it, especially considering that fat can lead to high cholesterol levels in the blood.

The truth is that the fats you eat only become a problem based on your carbohydrate intake. Otherwise, if you keep your carb intake in check as expected in the Atkins diet, then your body becomes and efficient fat burning machine, thereby fats do not end up causing poor health. In this way, the Atkins diet can be used to deal with Metabolic Syndrome.

Free Keto Diet Simplified Book

Hey! Want a free book? Check out my website and get

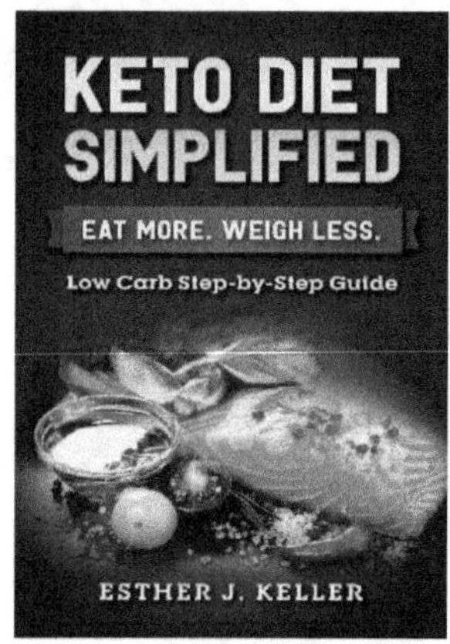

a FREE copy of **Keto Diet Simplified**.

Simply go to: www.EstherFitness.com

No strings attached. Promise.

Yours,

Leave a Review

If you found this short book was helpful at all or provided even a small insight that you took away, would you consider helping other people find this book by leaving this book an honest review? That'd mean a lot!

About the Author

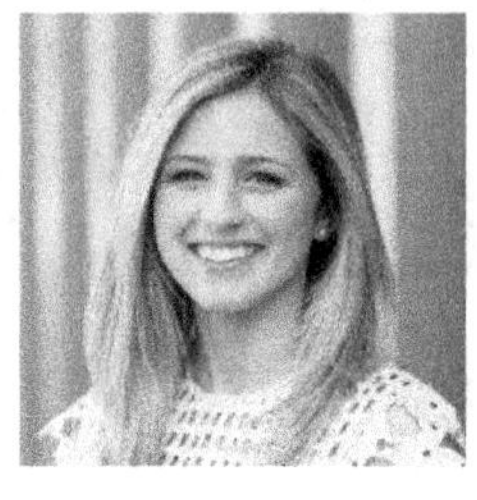

Esther Keller is a journalist by day and a runner by night. She loves long runs with her dog Russell and bike rides on chilly nights. She studied journalism at the University of Michigan and moved to Brooklyn upon graduating where she works as a fitness instructor. She loves reading, eating, exercising, hiking, sleeping and watching the Power Puff girls and New Girl.

Copyright